ALSO BY IAN K. SMITH, M.D.

The Take Control Diet
Dr. Ian Smith's Guide to Medical Websites
The Blackbird Papers: A Novel

THE FAT SMASH DIET

• The Last Diet You'll Ever Need •

Ian K. Smith, M.D.

Health Media Straegies, LLC New York City

AUTHOR'S NOTE: This book proposes a program of dietary and exercise

recommendations for the reader to follow. However, you should consult a qualified medical professional before starting this or any other weight reduction program. As with any diet or exercise program, if at any time you experience any discomfort, stop immediately and consult your physicians.

2006 Health Media Strategies, LLC Trade Paperback Edition

Published in the United States by Health Media Strategies.

Library of Congress Catalogue-in-Publication Data
Smith, Ian K., M.D.
The Fat Smash Diet: The Last Diet You'll Ever Need/Ian K. Smith, M.D.

ISBN 0-9776889-0-9

Printed in the United States of America

www.fatsmashdiet.com

9   8   7   6   5   4   3   2

First Edition

Book design by Sita Silva of FINN Creations

To Lynn Cherry, my beautiful aunt

May you lead a longer, healthier, and happier life now that you're 100 pounds lighter.

In the words of the great singer Barry White:

"I love you just the way you are."

THE FAT SMASH DIET
(Table of Contents)

NOTE FROM THE AUTHOR

Many of you have either seen or heard of my diet program on the popular VH1 show "Celebrity Fit Club." Over the past year I have received thousands of e-mails from viewers asking me to share with them the diet that I have put many Hollywood celebrities on with tremendous success. I want to get something clear right from the beginning. This is not a "celebrity" diet. This is a diet for EVERYONE. It is not based on gimmicks or false promises or fake science like a lot of other programs you'll find on the market. This is a nutritionally-sound, scientifically-based program that if followed correctly will deliver results even to those who have not succeeded on other diets.

With many years of experience working with tens of thousands of dieters, I have learned as much from the people who are trying to lose weight as they have learned from me. One of my biggest lessons—most dieters want a simple, easy-to-follow, realistic plan that does not require a tremendous amount of money or time. Dieters want to be able to eat reasonably, which means enjoying an ice cream cone or couple of chocolate chip cookies or slice of pizza every so often. It's ridiculous to think that people are going to go through the rest of their life without having a slice of cake for dessert or a drink of alcohol when socializing with family and friends. What I've learned is that if a meal plan includes a good percentage of "likeable" foods, then people are much more willing to stick to that program than a program that eliminates all of the "fun" foods and makes unrealistic dietary demands.

So I have decided to follow the advice and lessons I've gotten from thousands of dieters living all over the world. These pages are full of only relevant information as I have—excuse the pun—trimmed the fat to give you only the essentials that you will need to be successful. I have created The **FAT SMASH DIET** as an answer to all of the diet questions I've received over the years and the pleas from people who are simply fed up with being overweight. The **FAT SMASH DIET** is easy to follow, inexpensive, forgiving, and healthy. You will get as much out of it as you put into it. It has worked for not only Hollywood celebrities, but my friends and family members who couldn't believe they lost so much weight while still eating many of the foods they have always enjoyed.

You too can finally shed the weight and start feeling good about yourself both on the outside and inside. Remember, if you cheat, you're only cheating yourself. But if you follow the program and remain dedicated, you will be transformed into a new you and ready to take advantage of all the great things that life has to offer.

Enjoy!

Dr. Ian Smith

CHAPTER 1
The FAT SMASH Diet Philosophy

Diets don't fail people, rather people fail diets. The **FAT SMASH** Diet is a program that will never fail you if you open your mind to the great possibilities, believe in yourself, and give a full commitment. The **FAT SMASH** Diet is purposely designed to be a forgiving program that is as much about helping people make the necessary lifestyle changes to lead a healthier, happier, and longer life, as it is about getting rid of all of the extra weight that only increases your odds of developing devastating medical complications such as high blood pressure, diabetes, and heart disease. I'm a realist. Most people have a difficult time following diets to the letter of the law, slipping every once in a while when they can't resist the urges or when they've reached a plateau and feel like the weight is no longer coming off. The **FAT SMASH** Diet understands this and allows you to dial back into the program, by returning to phase I, getting back on course, then resuming the program where you left off.

The **FAT SMASH** Diet is specifically designed to be a 90-day program with four phases that will ultimately re-wire your body and its relationship to food and physical activity for the rest of your life. This is not about short-term fixes that will eventually fade and put you back at the beginning. Instead, this is about your life for the long term! At the end of the 90 days, you will have made small, but important adjustments not only in your food consumption, but your understanding and attitude towards food and the way you view the importance of physical activity in maintaining a healthy life. Each phase builds upon the previous phase like the levels of a pyramid that support the ones above it. The foundation and its integrity are what allow the peak to stand, so you must be careful in constructing the building blocks so that they might be as strong as possible to allow you to reach the top of your goals.

I have been shocked reading many diet books that say exercising is unnecessary or it's optional based on a dieter's preferences. The reason why I'm dumbfounded to read this is because one of the major reasons why so many people are overweight and obese and dying from preventable medical conditions such as heart disease is largely because we have become too sedentary of a society! There are numerous studies from the best researchers in the world that continuously show how important being physically active is not just for losing weight, but becoming healthier and protecting things like our blood vessels

Studies also show that those who incorporate a regular exercise program in their schedule will not only lose more weight faster, but will keep it off for longer periods of time. The problem that most people have is that they associate exercising with going to the gym and killing themselves for two hours, then dragging themselves home exhausted. That's not the exercise I'm talking about. Let's be realistic. It's not like you're training to become an Olympic gold medalist, right? What you need is a regular program of physical activity that will keep your heart rate up and your lungs working. This will also help with toning your muscles and keeping your joints active to help prevent certain illnesses like the dreaded arthritis. So for each phase I give you very simple exercise suggestions to help you on your journey of becoming healthier and slimmer. Choose those exercises that you like and try to find a partner who is willing to do them with you. Studies have also shown that those who are most successful at losing weight have some type of support system in place such as a weight-loss partner.

The **FAT SMASH** Diet is about smashing the bad habits and demons of the past and constructing a new and improved you now ready to take on new challenges and passions while fully enjoying the gift of life. Let's be perfectly clear. Diets are not magic. They are only blueprints. If you carefully follow the blueprint, then what you build can be magnificent. This is a blueprint that will help people trying to lose just 10 pounds as well as people trying to lose 200 pounds. I'm extremely proud of this program because it teaches the correct principles of eating healthy while at the same time allowing you to have a slice of cake or a couple of scoops of ice cream every now and again. Almost everything in life is about finding a balance and doing things in moderation. These are the underlying principles of The **FAT SMASH** Diet. You now are a SMASHER, so go SMASH IT!

Chapter 2
Phase I: DETOX (*9 days*)

This phase is ground zero, the beginning of the journey. The name detox pretty much says it all. For the next 9 days, you will eat fruits and veggies ONLY and clean your body and mind of impurities in a natural way without fasting or putting any "bad" toxins into your system. This is about purifying your body and blood and feeding them the nutrients, vitamins, and minerals that they so badly need. It's also about opening your mind and freeing it from the imprisonment of an unhealthy lifestyle that might be holding you back from reaching your peak. This is the first step towards a NEW YOU, so it's critical that you follow the principles of this phase and don't stray from the course.

Start by weighing yourself in the nude or a swimming suit the morning you start this phase, then don't weigh yourself again until the morning of day 10. Have someone photograph you in a bathing suit. Take three shots with your hands hanging freely by your sides—a frontal shot, one taken from the side, and the third from behind. Don't suck in your stomach or assume any unnatural poses. Just stand there and be real.

You need to record your healthy weight range, something that's indicated by your Body Mass Index (BMI). You can find this in the back appendix. This is the chart that doctors now use to determine what you should weigh for your particular height.

Surround yourself with positive energy and people who are supportive and respectful of your new journey. Reduce stressful occurrences in your life as stress only distracts you from your important missions and induces poor decisions. Try not to constantly think about food and weight! There's a lot more to life than food and worrying about the numbers on some inanimate scale. Take up a hobby and keep busy with the fun things in life. This will help the time fly and keep you energized. If your mind isn't in the right place, then you won't be able to lose the weight. Dieting is 50% mental. Don't forget that!

And remember, cheating is a decision, if that's the choice you make, you are only cheating yourself. Now let's start SMASHING!

NUMBER OF MEALS PER DAY: (4-5)

These meals are designed to be moderately-sized portions. Don't stuff your plate as if you won't be eating again. Now that you're eating more meals, you'll have less down time between meals, and you'll experience less hunger pains. Because you'll be eating every 3-4 hours, you don't need to eat so much at each meal. It's important that you understand this. Even if you're not hungry, it's **critical** that you don't skip meals. Just eat a lighter meal. Your body needs to get into a comfortable and reliable routine and it expects to be properly nourished at consistent time intervals.

QUANTITY OF FRUITS AND VEGGIES:

Eat the amount that fills you up. There is no limit and there's no counting calories. But even with this freedom, don't over eat! It's a bad habit and unnecessary. You'll be eating again soon enough. Portion control at all times!

MYTH:

If I skip meals or only eat once a day, I will lose weight because I'm eating less calories.

TRUTH:

The act of eating actually increases your metabolism, which helps you burn off the calories and lose weight. When you don't eat, your body goes into "starvation mode," which means your metabolism slows down tremendously and the calories that you do ingest are automatically stored as fat. The body does this, because fat is a great reserve of potential energy and can supply us in the future when this energy is needed. When you skip meals and "starve" yourself, the body doesn't know when it might see more food energy again, so it conserves and holds on to whatever it does see, and it stores it in the form of fat.

FOOD PREPARATION:

Foods are ONLY to be eaten raw, grilled, or steamed. You're allowed 3 tablespoons of low-fat dressing on your salads. If you're grilling the veggies, use minimal amount of virgin olive oil.

SAMPLE SCHEDULE:

Note: This is just a sample. You have to work out a schedule that fits your lifestyle, but keep in mind the spacing of the meals and the need to at least have 4 per day. For late night snacks, try sliced fruit or raw/steamed veggies like celery, carrots, cucumbers, broccoli, or asparagus.

8 am	Meal #1
11 am	Meal #2 *(heavy snack)*
2 pm	Meal #3
5 pm	Meal #4 *(light snack)*
7 pm	Meal #5
9 pm	Light Snack

DR. IAN'S TIP #1: Try frozen seedless grapes.
Put the grapes in the freezer, then
grab them as you like.
They're delicious and low in
calories!

DR. IAN'S TIP #2: Never eat within an hour and a half of
going to bed. Try going for at least a
20-25 minute walk after dinner
or participating in some type of
physical activity. This will help rev
up your metabolism and burn off
those calories before going to bed.
It also releases endorphins, special
chemicals in the body that make
you feel good!!

DR. IAN'S TIP #3: Eat foods high in fiber. Studies
have shown that fiber helps to make
you feel full longer, delay hunger
pains, reduce cholesterol levels,
reduce constipation, reduce the risk
of heart disease, and potentially
help prevent some intestinal
cancers. Dietary sources of fiber
include: whole grains, fruits,
vegetables, nuts, and seeds.

FOOD/DRINKS ALLOWED: *(Phase I)*

- All Fruits
- All Vegetables, except:
  NO white potatoes,
  NO avocados
- Good sources of protein:
  chick peas
  beans
  tofu
  lentils
- Brown Rice-2 cups of cooked
  rice per day
- 2 cups of low-fat or skim or
  soy milk per day
- Drink as much water as you like!
- Oatmeal-1 cup per day
- All herbs and spices
- 6 oz. low fat yogurt
  (2 times per day)
- 4 egg whites per day

FOOD/DRINKS NOT ALLOWED:
(Phase I)

- White Rice
- Meat
- Fish
- Bread-all types
- Raisins
- Nuts
- Dried or preserved sliced fruits
- Candy/Popcorn/Chips
- Ice Cream
- Alcohol
- Juice
- Soda
- Coffee
- Sports Drinks
- Milk Shakes
- Cappuccinos
- Café Latte

PHYSICAL ACTIVITY

At least 30 minutes of cardiovascular activity five days a week.

SAMPLE ACTIVITIES: AMOUNT OF CALORIES
(*Burned Per Hour*)

Pilates (light) 200

Pilates (moderate) 300

Elliptical machine (moderate) 300

Tennis: singles 350

Pilates (intense)................................400

Kickboxing . ...400 - 600

Dancing, Aerobic 420

Bicycle riding (moderate) 450

Power Walking (3mph) 450

Aerobics 450

Jogging (5 mph) 300

Swimming (active) 500

Hiking 500

Rowing (moderate effort) 550

Power Walking (intense effort)........................... 600

Basketball 700

Rowing (intense effort) 700

Running (11 to 30) 700

Jump Rope (moderate - 70 jumps / min) 700

Elliptical machine (intense) 700

Jump Rope (intense - 125 jumps / min) 850

Running (10 min mile) 850

Stair climbing (stadiums) 900

STRUCTURE: AT LEAST 30 minutes for 5 days a week. You can choose any five days you like. They don't have to be consecutive and can include all, part, or none of the weekend. It's also alright to do more days if you like. Anything over five is bonus!! Keep a simple journal of the type of physical activity you engaged in, the time of day you did it, and the amount of time you spent doing it.

SAMPLE SCHEDULE:

MON.	30 minutes - power walking (300 cal)
TUES.	OFF DAY
WED.	30 minutes - elliptical (350 cal)
THURS.	30 minutes - aerobics (225 cal)
FRI.	OFF DAY
SAT.	30 minutes - stair climbing (450 cal)
SUN.	30 minutes - cycling (225 cal)

DR IAN'S TIP #4: Try to get your workout done early in the morning. It's a great start to the day and it takes the pressure off of doing it later in the day, when you might be tired from a full day of work or busy with other life endeavors. Also, if you work out early in the morning, you can always do some type of physical activity at night for a bonus!

DR. IAN'S TIP #5: While it's faster and more organized to meet your physical activity component by working out in a gym, you don't have to belong to a gym to make this program work. Not everyone likes gyms and they can be costly. Try stair climbs or mini stadiums. Go up and down a flight of stairs of at least 10 steps. Up and back down is considered 1 trip. Try to do at least 10 trips within 30 minutes with 30-45 second rest periods between each trip. If you don't want to make noise in the house, go to the local high school track and use the bleachers. This is a GREAT work out and it doesn't cost anything.

DR. IAN'S TIP #6: CARDIO FAT BURNING

Work out with your heart rate in the fat-burning zone: 50-70% of maximal heart rate. Subtract your age from 220—this is your maximal heart rate. Then multiply that number by .50—this will give you the minimal heart rate you should maintain while performing your physical activity. Then take your maximal heart rate and multiply it by .70—this is the upper range for maximal fat burning.

EXAMPLE: (*40 year old person.*)

220 - 40 = 180 (maximal heart rate)

180 x .50 = 90 (lower limit of minimal fat-burning range)

180 x .70 = 126 (upper limit of maximal fat-burning range)

Range during exercise for maximal fat burning: 90-126 beats per minute

NOTE: THOSE WHO ARE BETTER CONDITIONED SHOULD WORK WITHIN THE RANGE 60-75% OF MAXIMAL HEART RATE

Chapter 3
Phase II: FOUNDATION
(*3 weeks*)

CONGRATULATIONS! You have gone through the most difficult part of the program: detoxification. Now that your body has detoxed and you have re-introduced the nourishing powers of fruits and vegetables to your diet, it's now time to start laying the foundation to a healthier way of eating and a healthier you.

The purpose of this phase is to re-introduce many of those foods you missed during detox, those very foods your body was craving to eat. At this point it's important to remember that this is about SMASHING those bad habits of the past and building good habits for the future. That means it's important to stick to the guidelines of the program with an understanding that you and your eating program are a work in progress. Now is not the time to undo all of the progress you've made in phase I, so some of the basic rules still apply: (1) do not over eat at any given sitting, but maintain the schedule of 4-5 smaller meals per day; (2) continue to eat as many fruits and vegetables as possible even though you are adding other foods to your diet; (3) remember, DON'T skip meals and stick as close as possible to the eating schedule that you've set up in phase I as this is what your body is now accustomed to following; (4) you MUST continue the physical activity portion of the program as this will be the best way that you continue to burn off those calories and SMASH the fat; (5) continue to stay away from heavily fried foods and fat-laden dressings that only add unnecessary calories and distribute bad fats in your blood.

Remember, we are building that pyramid and in order for the peak to remain towering beautifully in the sky, the blocks upon which it rests must remain strong and dependable. The blocks you put down in this phase are the most important as they comprise your FOUNDATION. Go SMASH it!

NUMBER OF MEALS PER DAY: (4-5)

It's EXTREMELY important that you eat at least 4 meals, because we are now adding more fun foods back in the diet and these fun foods pack a lot more calories than the fruits and vegetables of phase I. Eating multiple meals will reduce the time you're waiting between meals and continue to cut down on the hunger pains and cravings. Remember, it's all about smashing bad habits and building new ones. Setting a regular eating schedule is an important habit to develop! Maintain the smaller portions!

QUANTITY OF FRUITS AND VEGGIES:

As in the previous phase, there's no limit to the amount of fruits and veggies you can eat at each meal with the exception of avocados. Remember, this is a diet where you don't have to sit down with a calculator and figure out how many calories you're consuming. Let your hunger be your guide. Eat the fruits and veggies until the hunger is gone, but DON'T eat so much that you get up from the table feeling stuffed. This is essential. You will be re-energizing yourself in no more than a few hours, so don't overdo it in one sitting.

FOOD/DRINKS ALLOWED: *(Phase II)*

Vegetables:

- Bok choy
- Broccoli
- Collard greens
- Dark green leafy lettuce
- Kale
- Mesclun
- Romaine lettuce
- Spinach
- Watercress
- Acorn squash
- Butternut squash
- Carrots
- Pumpkin
- Sweet potatoes
- Black beans
- Black-eyed peas
- Chickpeas
- Kidney beans
- Lentils
- Corn
- Green peas

- Lima beans
- Artichokes
- Asparagus
- Bean sprouts
- Beets
- Brussel sprouts
- Cabbage
- Cauliflower
- Celery
- Cucumbers
- Eggplant
- Green beans
- Green/red peppers
- Mushrooms
- Okra
- Onions
- Parsnips
- Tomatoes
- Brown rice – 2 cups of cooked rice per day, every other day (if desired)
- Avocado –1/2 per day max
- 6 oz low fat yogurt (2 times per day)
- 4 egg whites per day

NEW NOTE: These are servings allowed per day and you can put it into the meal that you choose

MEATS *3-4 oz* size of a deck of playing cards	Chicken: baked without the skin (NO FRIED!!) Turkey: baked without the skin Ground beef: EXTRA lean or ground sirloin Sirloin steak Lamb
SEAFOOD	Halibut, Tuna, Salmon, Snapper, Striped Bass, etc. 3 oz (NO FRIED) Shrimp: 4 large Mussels: 3 oz Oysters: 6-12 Clams: 3
EGGS	Scrambled-1 per day Boiled-1 per day
MILK & CHEESE	2½ cups of low-fat, skim, or soy milk per day Cheese: 1 oz (about 1.5 slices)

➤➤

34

CEREALS
cold
unsweetened
1½ cups per day
hot
½ cup per day

Corn Flakes
Cheerios
Oatmeal
Farina/Cream of Wheat
Total
Bran Flakes
Life
Rice Crispies
Puffed rice
Puffed wheat
Shredded wheat
Wheaties
Special K
Chex

SWEETENERS

4 tsp of granulated sugar/day
(or sugar substitute)

SPICES & HERBS
as you like!

Salt (2 tsp per day)
Pepper (as you like)

➤➤

FLAVORINGS	2 tbsp of fat-free dressing per day Extra Virgin Olive Oil 1 tbsp per day 1 tbsp of fat-free mayo per day 2 packets of butter per day

DRINKS	1 10 oz cup of coffee per day
	3 cups of tea per day
	5 cups of club soda
	2 cans of diet soda per day
	1 cup of freshly squeezed
	     fruit juice per day (you can
	     divide this up into ½ cup
	     servings)
	Iced tea—sweetened only with 2
	     packets of sugar substitute
	Lemonade—made with real lemons
	     and 2 packets of sugar
	     substitute or 2 tsp. of table
	     sugar
	Flavored seltzer or tonic water
	     unlimited
	Unlimited tap or bottled water

FOOD/DRINKS NOT ALLOWED:
(Phase II)

- White rice
- White potatoes
- White bread/English muffins
- White pasta or Whole wheat pasta
- White flour
- Pastries/Donuts/Danish
- Cake
- Cookies
- Brownies
- Candy
- Ice Cream
- Potato Chips/Corn Chips/ Tortilla Chips/Popcorn
- Chocolate
- Bacon
- Sausage
- Alcohol

- Regular sodas
- Sweetened juices from a bottle or can
- Milk Shakes
- Frappuccinos
- Café Latte

TIPS:

-don't eat the same fish or meat twice in the same day

-try to separate the meats by at least a meal

-try to leave some of the food on your plate when
you get up from the table

-try to do some physical activity after eating dinner
(at least 20 minutes)

-only snack on fruits and veggies after dinner

-remember portion size, less is more!

PHYSICAL ACTIVITY:

Same program as phase I, except it's time to kick it up, because you're now eating a lot more calories, so you must increase everything by 10-15 %.
For example: if you walk for 30 minutes a day, now walk for 35.
If you walk a mile a day, now walk 1.1-1.2 miles.
Remember, do the cardio exercises in your heart ranges that were explained in phase I.
The more you do the better!
No lifting free weights!! (This will come)

SAMPLE SCHEDULE:

MON.	35 minutes - elliptical (408 cal)
TUES.	35 minutes - swimming (291 cal)
WED.	OFF DAY
THURS.	35 minutes - power walking (intense) (350 cal)
FRI.	OFF DAY
SAT.	35 minutes - aerobics (263 cal)
SUN.	35 minutes - jumping rope (408 cal)

Chapter 4
Phase III: CONSTRUCTION
(*4 weeks*)

Over the last two weeks, you have laid down a solid foundation for a healthier lifestyle that we will now continue to build on. This phase will add more variety to your diet, thus constructing an eating plan that will allow you to enjoy many of the foods you've enjoyed in the past. The difference, however, is that with your greater understanding of portion control and the importance of more fruits and vegetables in your diet, you can now enjoy some of those sweets you've missed in the past, but instead of eating five cookies, you'll be content with two. The first two phases should have instilled some important concepts that should guide your eating behaviors forever. Don't turn your back on all that you have learned and take up the old bad habits. Doing this will reverse the progress you've worked so hard to make.

Remember that you are now eating AT LEAST four

times a day, which means you don't have to fill your plate
to the rim, go back for seconds, or eat super-sized meals.
Your body is now accustomed to consistency: the regular
schedule of your eating times and the volume of food that
you're consuming at one sitting. Do the best that you can
not to disrupt this schedule, but if for some reason you
can't maintain it due to an extenuating circumstance like a
scheduling problem, then go back to it as soon as possible.
A short interruption will not throw you too far off course.
No dieter is perfect and at some time it is very likely
that you might slip. This is not uncommon. It happens
to almost everyone. If you face this situation, don't get
anxious. The **FAT SMASH** Diet is purposely designed
to forgive, not punish. Simply go back on phase I until
you've lost the weight that you had gained back. Once
you've lost that weight, go an extra day on phase I, then
back to phase III.

NUMBER OF MEALS PER DAY: (4-5)

QUANTITY OF FRUITS AND VEGGIES:

Let your hunger be your guide. Eat enough that
satisfies, not enough that stuffs. Remember these foods are
most nutritious when they're eaten raw, steamed, grilled or
baked. Frying is not permitted as this adds extra calories
and destroys the nutrients buried in the food.

FOOD/DRINKS ALLOWED: *(Phase III)*

Vegetables:

- Bok choy
- Broccoli
- Collard greens
- Dark green leafy lettuce
- Kale
- Mesculin
- Romaine lettuce
- Spinach
- Watercress
- Acorn squash
- Butternut squash
- Carrots
- Pumpkin
- Sweet potatoes
- Black beans
- Black-eyed peas
- Chickpeas
- Kidney beans
- Lentils
- Corn

- Green peas
- Lima beans
- Artichokes
- Asparagus
- Bean sprouts
- Beets
- Brussel sprouts
- Cabbage
- Cauliflower
- Celery
- Cucumbers
- Eggplant
- Green beans
- Green/red peppers
- Mushrooms
- Okra
- Onions
- Parsnips
- Tomatoes
- Brown rice-2 cups of cooked rice per day, every other day (if desired)
- Avocado-1/2 per day max

Cold unsweetened 1½ cups per day

Hot ½ cup per day

- Corn Flakes
- Cheerios
- Oatmeal
- Farina/Cream of Wheat
- Total
- Bran Flakes
- Life
- Rice Crispies
- Puffed rice
- Puffed wheat
- Shredded wheat
- Wheaties
- Special K
- Chex
- 4 tsp of granulated sugar/day
- Salt (2 tsp per day)
- Pepper (as you like)

- 2 tbsp of fat-free dressing per day
- Extra Virgin Olive Oil
- 1 tbsp per day
- 1 tbsp of fat-free mayo per day
- 2 packets of butter per day
- 1 10 oz cup of regular coffee per day
- 3 cups of tea per day
- 5 cups of club soda
- 2 cans of diet soda per day
- Iced tea—sweetened only with 2 packets of sugar substitute
- Lemonade—made with real lemons and 2 packets of sugar substitute or 2 tsp of table sugar
- Flavored seltzer or tonic water unlimited
- Unlimited tap or bottled water!

NEW

- 2 cups of freshly squeezed fruit juice per day (you can divide this up throughout the day as you like)

NEW

NOTE: These are servings allowed per day and you can put it into the meal that you choose; meat serving is now larger.

MEATS *5 oz* size of a deck and a half of playing cards	Chicken: baked without the skin (NO FRIED!!) Turkey: baked without the skin Ground beef: EXTRA lean or ground sirloin Sirloin steak Lamb Turkey Sausage-1 link
SEAFOOD	Halibut, Tuna, Salmon, Snapper, Striped Bass, etc. 3 oz (NO FRIED) Shrimp: 4 large Mussels: 3 oz Oysters: 6-12 Clams: 3
EGGS	Scrambled-2 per day Boiled-2 per day (Whites only-4 per day)
MILK & CHEESE	3 cups of low-fat, skim, or soy milk per day Cheese: 1.3 oz (about 2 slices)

*new
PASTA

Whole wheat pasta: 1 cup per day
Whole wheat/Whole grain bread:
4 thin slices per day

*new
DESSERTS

the serving size
for the cookies is
approximately
the size of
a silver dollar
(*e.g. an oreo*)

Note: *These are servings per day;*
one dessert per day at any time of
your choosing.

3 chocolate chip

4 gingersnaps

2 oatmeal raisin

2 peanut butter

2 whole Graham Crackers

1 scoop of low-fat ice cream

FOOD/DRINKS NOT ALLOWED:
(Phase III)

- White rice
- White potatoes
- White bread/English muffins
- White pasta
- White flour
- Pastries/Donuts/Danish
- Cake
- Brownies
- Candy
- Potato Chips/Corn Chips/Tortilla Chips/Popcorn
- Bacon
- Sausage
- Alcohol
- Regular sodas
- Milk Shakes
- Frappuccinos
- Café Latte

PHYSICAL ACTIVITY:

Same program as phase II, except it's time to kick it up, because you're now eating a lot more calories, so you must increase everything by 25 %.

For example: if you walk for 35 minutes a day, now walk for 45 mins.

If you walk 1.1 miles a day, now walk 1.4 miles a day

Remember, do the cardio exercises in your heart range that was explained in Tip #6 of phase I.

Light free weights optional, but better to do them in the next phase.

SAMPLE SCHEDULE:

MON.	OFF DAY
TUES.	45 minutes - aerobics (338 cal)
WED.	45 minutes - elliptical (525 cal)
THURS.	OFF DAY
FRI.	45 minutes - basketball, full court (525 cal)
SAT.	45 minutes - swimming (375 cal)
SUN.	45 minutes - stair climbing (675 cal)

Chapter 5
Phase IV: THE TEMPLE
(*for life*)

The fact that you've made it to this phase means that you have achieved tremendous success. This is no small feat. Be proud of yourself! You have **detoxed** your body, laid a solid **foundation** for a healthier way of living, and **constructed** a routine of good habits that will guide you throughout your life. All of this is like building a sacred temple, something to admire, respect, and honor. But like any beautiful structure, there's also maintenance involved to keep it clean and shiny. Every once in a while there will be the need for minor repairs, and that's expected. The key, however, is to avoid the need for major fixes. This is where you are on The **FAT SMASH** Diet. Now that you've built the temple of good eating behaviors and a physical activity program, you can admire and appreciate it, but also be prepared for minor tweaks as you go along. Remember that life is constantly evolving.

where the repairs need to be done or when. Maybe you've started eating too many sweets or increased the portions beyond the appropriate sizes. Some people will start slacking off on the physical activity regimen and will notice the weight slowly starting to pile back on. Don't get upset or frustrated. These are not major problems and can be addressed very easily. That's the beauty of The **FAT SMASH** Diet. The important part here is to identify the exact location of the leak in the roof and quickly use the necessary material to fix it. If you notice that you've gained back 10-15 % of the weight that you had lost earlier, then simply leave the temple (phase IV), go back to detox (phase I) until you've lost that weight again, then return to the temple being mindful of your portions and keeping up your physical activity so that you can enjoy what you've worked so hard to build.

In this last phase, there are some food and beverage additions for you that will complete your eating program. Since they've been absent from your diet for the last eight weeks, you can better appreciate them, but it's important to follow the guidelines and not overindulge. Remember, at this stage of the diet, you have SMASHED the bad habits and developed good, healthy habits through hard work and determination. This healthier way of living can sustain you forever.

NEW NOTE: The foods from all of the previous phases are allowed in this phase. Now you have more to add below. Enjoy, but remember, *PORTION CONTROL!*

BREAKFAST	Bacon: 4 strips per week Sausage: 2 links per week 6 four inch pancakes per week (whole wheat is better) 1 6-inch waffle per week
LUNCH & DINNER	2 slices of cheese pizza with any toppings-twice a week white rice-2 servings a week (but brown is still better) 1 white baked potato a week (but sweet potato is still better) 2 small servings of french fries per week
DRINKS	2 8-oz cups of soda per week (diet soda is much better) 2-3 beers per week (preferably not at one sitting) 3 glasses of wine per week (preferably not at one sitting) 3 8 oz cafe lattes per week (try using fat-free milk) 1 12 oz milk shake per week

PHYSICAL ACTIVITY:

By this point you should be in a comfortable routine. Exercise 5 times a week for 1 intense hour. It's very important to change your workout routine as your body can quickly become accustomed to your exercise schedule and stop burning the calories.

Also, start lifting light free weights under supervision. This will help build up your lean muscle mass. You should lift weights at least twice a week, working on your different body parts. You can do this right at home with dumbbells. But you should make sure you have been trained on the proper lifting techniques before attempting.

Your physical activity plan is ESSENTIAL for you to develop the complete package. It will only boost the results you obtain on the diet!

Chapter 6
BUSTING THROUGH THE PLATEAU

Almost everyone over the course of a diet hits a plateau, a point where they can't seem to lose anymore weight despite their previous success. This is what I call the critical point. It's critical, because unfortunately, most people get frustrated and disappointed and quit. DON'T DO THAT! Plateaus are very natural and happen for a good reason. The body is an extremely clever machine and while we think that we can fool it, we can only do so for short periods of time at best. The body becomes accustomed to your new way of eating and your exercise regimen and decides that it is not going to keep burning calories by shedding fat. Believe it or not, that's an important protective feature of how our bodies operate. Imagine if you were stuck on a cold mountain with no way of getting food or water for a prolonged period of time. The body works to conserve your fat—the source of energy—as long as possible so that you can last without food and water for a prolonged period of time. Well, it's that feature that kicks in when you've been doing so well losing weight.

But there is a way to bust through this "standstill point" and it requires patience and determination. First, each time you exercise, increase it by 20% and do this for 9 days. For example, if you normally walk for 60 minutes during your exercise time, walk for 72 minutes instead. If you normally walk 2 miles at a time, walk 2.4 miles. At the same time, decrease the amount of calories you consume by eating smaller portions. This way, you're attacking the problem from both ends.

Another method is to change your diet altogether. Sometimes you have to "shock" the system to get it going. So go back to an earlier phase like I or II or a combination of them and stay there for 7 days. You can play with the combination as you like, but the idea is to do something different than what you've been doing. You should also change your exercise program. Try to do a different exercise. If you spend most of your time walking, then try doing stairs or playing a sport. Don't decrease your time, just switch up the activity.

The bottom line is that in order to bust through the plateau, you must shake your body out of its comfort zone. Do this for 7-9 days and this should get you through it. There's no universal solution that works for everyone, but I have found these strategies to be very effective for most dieters whom I have helped over the years.

Chapter 7
TASTY RECIPES

Most recipes provided by Big City Chefs: 1-866-321-CHEF **www.bigcitychefs.com**

NOTE: Look at the serving size for the different recipes. In many cases it's 4 or more for that particular recipe, which means you are not to eat all of it. You are still ONLY to have 1 serving size per meal at most! Remember, this is about portion control. You are eating more meals per day, which means each meal MUST be smaller or you'll be packing on too many calories!

SAMPLE SCHEDULE:

MON.	60 minutes - elliptical (700 cal)
TUES.	60 minutes - swimming (500 cal)
WED.	OFF DAY
THURS.	60 minutes - power walking (intense) (600 cal)
FRI.	OFF DAY
SAT.	60 minutes - aerobics (450 cal)
SUN.	60 minutes - jumping rope, 70 jumps /min (700 cal)

PHASE I | Sample Recipes

LIST BREAKFAST GOOD HABITS

_____
_____
_____
_____
_____
_____
_____
_____
_____
_____

LIST BREAKFAST BAD HABITS

_____
_____
_____
_____
_____
_____
_____
_____
_____
_____
_____
_____

Breakfast | (*phase I*)

Recipes on the go!

- ½ cup oatmeal
  1 cup of raspberries
  1 cup low-fat milk

- ½ cantaloup
  6 oz cup low-fat yogurt
  1 cup of fresh orange juice

- 4 egg whites
  ½ red grapefruit
  1 cup of low-fat milk

Lunch | (*phase I*)

(Green Bean Salad)

Serves : 4-6

1	lb green beans, fresh and trimmed
10	halved cherry tomatoes
1	yellow sweet pepper, seeded and julienned
½	cup chopped green pepper
¼	cup chopped fresh parsley

Dressing :

1	tsp of Dijon mustard
¼	cup of olive oil
¼	tsp freshly ground pepper
¼	cup of fresh lemon juice
⅛	tsp of salt

DIRECTIONS

Wash green beans thoroughly. Drop the green beans in a sauce pan of boiling water. Cook until slightly crisp.

Drain off water and let beans cool.

Add tomatoes, peppers, parsley.

To make dressing, take small bowl combine mustard, oil, and lemon juice. Stir well.

Then add pepper and salt and stir again.

Lightly pour the dressing over the salad, then toss, then transfer to serving bowl, cover, and refrigerate until well chilled for at least an hour.

(Vigorous Vegetable Soup)

Serves : 4

1   chopped medium zucchini
1   cup of chopped mushrooms
1   medium onion
7   large carrots
4   celery stalks
1   sprig of rosemary
1   tsp of dried thyme
1   bay leaf
¼   tsp crushed red pepper flakes
1   (*10 ounce*) package frozen
    green peas, thawed
3   (14.5 ounce) can low fat,
    low sodium beef broth
    (or vegetable broth)
3   cups water

DIRECTIONS

Place the zucchini, mushrooms, onion, carrots, celery, and peas into a large pot with the water, broth, and spices.

Bring to a boil, then let it simmer for 1 to 1½ hours or until carrots are tender.

Remove the bay leaf and rosemary sprig before serving.

(Carrot Soup)

Serves : 4

10   carrots

5   cups (40 oz) of vegetable
      broth or beef broth

1   small onion, chopped

3   tbsp of curry

¼   cup brown rice (optional)

1   tbsp minced ginger

2   cloves garlic

     Parsley

     Bay leaves

1   tsp butter

     salt and pepper

DIRECTIONS

Melt butter in medium skillet. Add carrots and onion and sauté until soft (approx. 10-15 minutes).

Next add salt, pepper, broth, parsley, bay leaves, and rice and boil for 30-40 minutes.

Remove parsley and bay leaves, then pour mix in a blender and purée.

Serve hot or cold.

Dinner | (*phase I*)

Lentils with Grilled Mushrooms, Asparagus, and Asparagus Broth

Serves : 4

- 3 cups lentils, cooked
- 2 cups mushrooms
- 1 tsp garlic, minced
- 1 cup asparagus, steamed and chopped
- 2 tbsp fresh basil, cut into chiffonade (thin strips)

  salt and pepper to taste

For asparagus broth :
- 3 tbsp olive oil
- 3 cups vegetable broth
- 2 cloves garlic
- ½ cup asparagus ends, roughly chopped (*use leftover woody ends of stems that are not used above*)
- ¼ cup carrot, onion, celery, chopped
- 2 tbsp white wine
- 2 tsp olive oil
- 1 bay leaf

  basil stems

  salt and pepper to taste

DIRECTIONS

To make asparagus broth :
Heat olive oil over medium heat and sweat carrots, onions, celery and garlic cloves, approximately 2 minutes.
Add white wine and cook for 1 minute. Add asparagus ends, broth, bay leaf, and basil stems. Reduce heat and simmer for 20 minutes. Strain and set aside.

Toss mushrooms with 2 tablespoons of olive oil and grill on medium heat for 2 minutes per side (you may alternately oven roast them on a baking sheet for 10 minutes at 400° F). Let mushrooms cool, then slice. Heat 1 tbsp olive oil in a sauté pan over high heat, add garlic and briefly sweat until aromas are released. Add lentils, mushrooms, and asparagus and cook for 1 minute over high heat. Add asparagus broth and bring to a simmer. Heat through until all ingredients are hot. Remove from the heat, add fresh basil, season to taste with salt and pepper, and serve.

NUTRITIONAL INFORMATION:

Per Serving (excluding unknown items): 417 Calories; 14g Fat (29.2% calories from fat); 20g Protein; 56g Carbohydrate; 16g Dietary Fiber; 2mg Cholesterol; 1235mg Sodium. Exchanges: 3 Grain(Starch); 1 Lean Meat; 1 Vegetable; 3 Fat.

(Corn Salad)

Serves: 4

½   pound of sweet yellow corn

1   cup grape tomatoes, cut in half

1   medium onion, chopped

3   portobello mushrooms, chopped

⅓   cup balsamic vinegar

⅓   cup olive oil

4   tsp water

    salt and pepper to taste

½   cup fresh parsley, chopped

½   cup chives, chopped (optional)

1   bell pepper, chopped

    pinch of brown or white sugar

¼   to ½ pound of baby lettuce

DIRECTIONS

Marinate the mushrooms for 45 minutes in vinegar, olive oil, water, and sugar.

While mushrooms marinate, mix corn, tomatoes, lettuce, pepper, parsley, chives, salt and pepper in large bowl.

Drizzle the mushroom vinaigrette over salad or keep to the side and dip.

(Grilled Vegetable Platter)

Serves: 4

2   yellow sweet peppers

2   red sweet peppers

3   zucchini

3   squash

18 asparagus

4   tomatoes

Dressing (*makes about 1 cup*)

¾   cup olive oil

3   tbsp balsamic vinegar

2   cloves minced garlic

1   tsp fresh lemon juice

pinch of dried basil

pinch of dried oregano

salt and freshly ground pepper

DIRECTIONS

Slice the vegetables and grill them to your preference.

Cook peppers till charred.

Cook zucchini and squash-about 4 mins on each side; Asparagus-5 mins.

Cook tomatoes-about 3 mins on each side.

Drizzle vegetables lightly with dressing.

Chilled Asparagus with Rosemary and Lemon Vinaigrette

Serves : 4-6

30	asparagus spears, peeled and tough ends trimmed
2	medium garlic cloves
2	tbsp fresh rosemary, chopped
2	tbsp red wine vinegar
½	cup of extra virgin olive oil
2	tsp fresh lemon juice
	light salt and pepper to taste
1	tsp low-fat mayonnaise

DIRECTIONS

Take a small bowl and combine lemon juice,
rosemary, garlic, and mayonnaise. Whisk in the
olive oil slowly to create creamy sauce. Season
with salt and pepper.

Trim tough white ends off of the asparagus.
Bring large sauté pan of water to a boil and
add asparagus. Boil until tender. Remove the
asparagus, then shock it in ice water (a gallon of
water and three ice trays) for about 2 minutes to
stop the asparagus from cooking.

Drain asparagus again and place on paper towels to
pat dry. Then arrange the asparagus on a serving
platter. Cover and refrigerate until completely
chilled. (About 1 hour).

When it's time to serve, pour vinaigrette evenly
over the asparagus.

(Tasty Tomatoes)

Serves : 4-6

4   medium tomatoes

2   tsp of finely chopped chives

4   tbsp of grated parmesan cheese

3   tbsp of low-fat mayonnaise

1 ½   tsp of Dijon mustard

     light salt and pepper

DIRECTIONS

Preheat the oven to 375° F.

Cut tomatoes in half and place the cut side facing up on a baking tray.

In a bowl, stir the topping: chives, mayonnaise, mustard, salt and pepper, and 2 tablespoons of parmesan cheese.
Once the topping is nicely mixed, scoop out small amounts with a spoon and place on top of the tomatoes.

Take the rest of the cheese that hasn't been used and sprinkle on top. Then bake for 10 minutes or until the tomatoes are hot. Once this is done, then quickly put in the broiler to really get the topping brown and hot.

Serve hot.

WHAT WAS EASY IN PHASE I

WHAT WAS DIFFICULT IN PHASE I

PHASE II | Sample Recipes

LIST NEW FOODS THAT YOU'VE COME TO LIKE

Breakfast | (*phase II*)

Recipes on the go!

- 1 cup bran cereal
  1 cup low-fat milk
  1 medium banana
  1 cup orange juice

- 1½ cup puffed wheat
  1 cup low-fat milk
  ¼ cantaloupe

- 2 boiled eggs
  6 oz plain yogurt
  1 cup low-fat milk

Lunch | (*phase II*)

Kidney Beans with Sautéed Shrimp and Asparagus

Serves : 4

3   cups kidney beans, cooked
    and drained.
12 oz raw shrimp, peeled and deveined

marinade for shrimp :
2   tbsp fresh lemon juice
2   tsp fresh thyme, chopped
4   tbsp basil, chiffonade
1   clove garlic
1   tbsp extra virgin olive oil
    salt and pepper to taste
1   tbsp olive oil
2   tbsp white wine
2   cups asparagus, steamed and chopped
2   cups vegetable stock
1   tbsp each fresh basil and
    thyme, chopped
    salt and pepper to taste

DIRECTIONS

Combine marinade ingredients, add shrimp, and let stand in refrigerator for 20 minutes.

Drain marinade.

Heat 1 tbsp olive oil in a sauté pan over high heat and cook shrimp for 2 minutes per side.

Add garlic and briefly sweat until aromas are released.

Add kidney beans and white wine and cook for 1 minute over high heat.

Add stock, bring to a simmer, and add asparagus.

Heat through until all ingredients are hot and shrimp is a white, opaque color.

Remove from the heat, add fresh herbs, season to taste with salt and pepper, and serve.

NUTRITIONAL INFORMATION:
Per Serving (excluding unknown items): 429 Calories; 11g Fat (23.0% calories from fat); 33g Protein; 49g Carbohydrate; 12g Dietary Fiber; 131mg Cholesterol, 945mg Sodium. Exchanges: 3 Grain(Starch); 3 Lean Meat; 1/2 Vegetable; 0 Fruit; 2 Fat.

Greek Vegetable Stew with Garbanzo Beans

Serves : 4

2 cups garbanzo beans, cooked
2 cups onion, diced
1½ cups green bell pepper, diced
2 cups mushrooms, sliced
2 cups artichoke hearts, sliced
   (can use frozen or canned if
   fresh not available)
1 tbsp olive oil
1 tsp cumin
1 pinch cinnamon
2 tbsp garlic, minced
1 ½ qt vegetable broth
3 cups roma tomatoes, chopped
   salt and pepper to taste
1 tbsp lemon juice
⅓ cup kalamata olives, pitted and sliced
1 tbsp oregano, chopped
2 tbsp mint, chopped
2 tbsp dill, chopped
½ cup feta, crumbled

DIRECTIONS

In saucepan, heat olive oil over high heat and add onion, green pepper, mushrooms, artichokes, cumin and cinnamon, and cook until golden brown, approximately 5 minutes, stirring occasionally.

Add garlic and stir, cooking for 20-30 seconds until the aromas are released.

Add stock and simmer for 15 minutes.

Add tomatoes and garbanzo beans, simmering for an additional 5 minutes.

Remove from heat, add olives, mint and dill, and serve in bowls, garnished with crumbled feta.

NUTRITIONAL INFORMATION:

Per Serving (excluding unknown items): 652 Calories; 22g Fat (28.7% calories from fat); 26g Protein; 96g Carbohydrate; 17g Dietary Fiber; 20mg Cholesterol; 3071mg Sodium. Exchanges: 4 Grain(Starch); 1 Lean Meat; 5 1/2 Vegetable; 0 Fruit; 4 Fat.

Seafood Gumbo with Brown Rice

Serves : 4

1	lb raw seafood, in any combination of fish or shrimp
⅓	cup whole wheat flour
⅓	cup olive oil
1	cup onion
3	cloves garlic
1	cup celery
1	cup green pepper
3	tbsp file powder
1	tsp cayenne pepper
1 ½	quarts vegetable stock
1 ½	cups okra
1	cup tomatoes
1	tbsp each fresh oregano, basil, thyme
½	lb seafood sausage, cooked and sliced (optional) – available at specialty markets
	salt and pepper to taste
8	oz brown rice
1	quart water
	salt to taste

DIRECTIONS

Heat olive oil over medium-low heat and add flour. Stir into a paste and cook for several minutes until a rich nutty brown. This mixture is called a "roux."

Add diced onion, garlic, celery and green pepper to roux and cook for approximately 2 minutes, stirring constantly. Roux will cling to vegetables.

Add seafood and cook for approximately 3 minutes. Add file powder and cayenne powder. Add chicken stock and bring mixture to a simmer for ten minutes, stirring constantly.

Add okra and tomatoes (and sausage if using) and cook for 2 minutes.

Season to taste with salt.

To make brown rice, bring rice, 1 quart of water, and salt to boil in an uncovered pot. Then reduce heat to low, cover, and simmer for approximately 45 minutes.

My Mother's Yummy Teriyaki Green Beans

Serves : 4

1   lb bag of frozen green beans

2   tbps of olive oil

¼   cup of MCcormick Grill Mates
      teriyaki grilling sauce

1   cup Kikkoman stir fry sauce

3   tbsp of House of Tsang
      classic stir fry sauce

2   shakes of worcestershire sauce

2   shakes of soy sauce

2   shakes of Kikkoman
      teriyaki sauce

DIRECTIONS

Heat oil until very hot.
Drop frozen beans into oil and turn immediately
to coat beans with oil.

Add the remaining ingredients and stir until well
coated.

Cook on low until tender.

Season to taste.

Chopped Vegetable Salad

Serves : 4-6

2   cucumbers, peeled and sliced
2   cups grape tomatoes, sliced in half
2   scallions, finely chopped (optional)
1   bell pepper, chopped
1   cup fresh green beans
½   cup of cooked corn
2   carrots, chopped
2   tsp chives, minced

Dressing :
⅓   cup of balsamic vinegar
½   tsp garlic
⅓   cup of extra virgin oil
    salt and pepper to taste

DIRECTIONS

Mix well the cucumbers, tomatoes, scallions, pepper, beans, corn, carrots, and chives in a large bowl.

In smaller bowl, mix oil, vinegar, salt, and pepper to taste. Stir well.

Pour dressing over vegetables. Chill for fifteen minutes in refrigerator, then serve.

Dinner | (*phase II*)

Garbanzo Beans with Chicken, Broccoli, and Tomato Broth

Serves : 4-6

3   cups garbanzo beans, cooked
2   boneless, skinless chicken breasts, julienned

Marinade :

2   tbsp fresh lemon juice
2   tsp fresh oregano, chopped
4   tbsp fresh basil, cut into chiffonade (thin strips)
1   clove garlic
1   tbsp extra virgin olive oil
    salt and pepper to taste
1   tbsp olive oil
2   cups broccoli, steamed and chopped

Tomato Broth :

3   Roma tomatoes, roughly chopped
1   tbsp olive oil
1   bunch basil stems (after leaves have been removed for marinade)
1   bay leaf
3   cups chicken broth
2   garlic cloves, whole
¼   cup each of carrot, onion, celery, chopped
1   tbsp white wine
    salt and pepper to taste

DIRECTIONS

To make tomato broth, heat olive oil over medium
heat and sweat carrots, onions, celery and garlic
cloves, approximately 2 minutes.

Add white wine and cook for 1 minute.

Add tomatoes, broth, bay leaf, and basil stems.
Reduce heat and simmer for 20 minutes.

Strain and set aside.

Combine marinade ingredients, add chicken, and let
stand in refrigerator for 20 minutes. Drain marinade.

Heat 1 tbsp olive oil in a sauté pan over high heat
and cook chicken until fully cooked (test one piece
by cutting into it).
Add garlic and briefly sweat until aromas are released.

Add garbanzo beans and cook for 1 minute over high
heat. Add tomato broth, bring to a simmer, and add
broccoli. Heat through until all ingredients are hot.

Remove from the heat, add fresh herbs, season to
taste with salt and pepper, and serve.

NUTRITIONAL INFORMATION:
Per Serving (excluding unknown items) : 486 Calories; 15g Fat
(28.9% calories from fat); 41g Protein; 45g Carbohydrate; 7g
Dietary Fiber; 68mg Cholesterol; 1724mg Sodium. Exchanges: 2
Grain(starch); 4 1/2 Lean Meat; 1/2 Vegetables;
0 Fruit; 2 1/2 Fat.

(Roasted Sea Bass)

Serves : 4

4	sea bass fillets without the skin
3	tbsp chopped fresh parsley
2	tbsp drained capers (optional)
2	tbsp minced fresh basil
1	tsp Dijon mustard
1	tbsp fresh lemon juice
3	tbsp extra-virgin olive oil
1	garlic clove, chopped
	salt and freshly ground pepper
½	cup fresh bread crumbs
	(optional for Phase II)

DIRECTIONS

Preheat oven to 350° F.

Take a small bowl and mix bread crumbs, clove, mustard, salt, parsley, capers, and pepper.

Put 3 tablespoons of olive oil in a frying pan and sauté the sea bass for about 5 minutes on each side.

Apply the bread crumb mix to the fish and make sure it adheres. Place the on a rack within a roasting pan.

Cook to your preference.

WHAT WAS EASY IN PHASE II

_____

_____

_____

_____

_____

_____

_____

_____

_____

_____

WHAT WAS DIFFICULT IN PHASE II

_____

_____

_____

_____

_____

_____

_____

_____

_____

_____

_____

_____

PHASE III | Sample Recipes

LIST ALL GOOD HABITS LEARNED IN PHASES I & 2

_____

_____

_____

_____

_____

_____

_____

_____

_____

_____

_____

_____

_____

_____

_____

_____

_____

_____

_____

_____

_____

_____

_____

_____

_____

_____

Breakfast | (*phase III*)

Recipes on the go!

- 1 English muffin, toasted
  2 tsp peanut butter
  ¾ cup plain low-fat yogurt
  ¾ cup blackberries

- ½ bagel, toasted
  4 egg whites
  1 cup fresh orange juice

- 2 eggs, scrambled
  1 English muffin
  1 tsp butter or margarine
  1 cup fresh orange juice

Country Breakfast Patty
with Oatmeal and Side of Fruit

Serves : 4

8	ounces ground turkey
2	eggs
2	tablespoons red bell pepper, chopped
2	tablespoons yellow onion – diced
1	teaspoon fresh thyme – chopped
	salt and pepper to taste
1	tablespoon olive oil
½	cup dry instant oats
1	cup skim milk
1	cup strawberries – sliced

DIRECTIONS

Combine ground turkey, eggs, bell pepper, onion, thyme, and salt and pepper, and form into 4 patties.

Sauté patties in olive oil until cooked through and golden brown on both sides, approximately 3 minutes on each side, depending on thickness of patties.

Cook oats in milk according to package instructions.

Serve patty with side of sliced strawberries and oatmeal.

NUTRITIONAL INFORMATION:

Per Serving (excluding unknown items): 224 Calories; 11g Fat (46.1% calories from fat); 17g Protein; 13g Carbohydrate; 2g Dietary Fiber; 132mg Cholesterol; 223mg Sodium. Exchanges: 1/2 Grain(Starch); 2 Lean Meat; 0 Vegetable; 0 Fruit; 0 Non-Fat Milk; 1 Fat.

Tropical Fruit Salad
with side of Turkey Sausage

Serves : 4

2   Large Turkey Sausages

⅓   *cup each* :

Pineapple, peeled, cored, and

cut into spears

Mango, pitted peeled, and

cut into spears

Papaya, pitted, peeled, and

cut into spears

Banana, sliced

Strawberries, sliced

Kiwi, peeled and sliced

Mint leaves for garnish

DIRECTIONS

To make fruit salad, combine fruit and toss.

Cook turkey sausage in a 400 degree oven for approximately ten minutes or until done.

Cut sausages into halves and serve with fruit salad, garnished with mint leaf.

NUTRITIONAL INFORMATION:

Per Serving (excluding unknown items): 185 Calories; 11g Fat (52.8% calories from fat); 9g Protein; 14g Carbohydrate; 2g Dietary Fiber; 45mg Cholesterol; 382mg Sodium. Exchanges: 1 Lean Meat; 1 Fruit; 1 1/2 Fat.

Poached Eggs and Spinach on English Muffin with Tomato-Mint Coulis

Serves : 4

8	large eggs
2	cups spinach, steamed
4	whole wheat English muffins
2	tsp distilled white vinegar
2	roma tomatoes, roughly chopped
1	tsp olive oil
1	tsp red wine vinegar
½	clove garlic, minced
1	tbsp onion, roughly chopped
1	tbsp mint, chopped
	salt and pepper to taste

DIRECTIONS

To make the coulis :
In a saucepan, heat olive oil over medium heat and
sweat garlic and onion until translucent. Add
tomatoes and cook for 10 minutes. Add vinegar
and simmer for an additional two minutes. Season
to taste with salt and pepper, remove from heat,
and puree in food processor until smooth. Add
fresh mint.

Heat one gallon of water in a stockpot with white
vinegar to a low simmer.

Toast English muffins.

Carefully crack eggs directly into water and vinegar
mixture, and let cook for 4 minutes.

Remove with slotted spoon.

Spoon warm spinach over muffins, and top with eggs.

NUTRITIONAL INFORMATION:

Per Serving (excluding unknown items): 311 Calories; 13g Fat (35.9%
calories from fat); 19g Protein; 31g Carbohydrate; 5g Dietary Fiber;
1 1/2 Lean Meat; 1/2 Vegetable; 1 Fat; 0 Other Carbohydrates.

Mushroom, Pepper, and Provolone Frittata with Macerated Fresh Berries

Serves : 4

1   red bell pepper, diced and
    sautéed in olive oil
1   cup mushrooms, sliced and
    sautéed in olive oil
4   large eggs
14 egg whites
4   thin slices of provolone
1   tbsp parmesan
1   tsp olive oil
    salt and pepper to taste
2   cups blueberries,
    strawberries,
    raspberries, and blackberries
1   tbsp granulated sugar substitute
    (splenda recommended)
1   tbsp lemon juice

DIRECTIONS

Sauté red pepper and mushrooms in ½ tablespoon of olive oil over high heat for about 2 minutes or until softened. Whisk together whole eggs and egg whites, and season to taste with salt and pepper.

In a separate pan, heat remaining olive oil over high heat and add eggs, stirring every minute for a total of approximately 5 minutes or until eggs are set.

Layer vegetables, provolone, and parmesan on top of omelet and place in a 500 degree oven or under broiler for 2 minutes.

Cut into wedges and serve hot.

To macerate berries, toss berries, sugar substitute, and lemon juice.

Serve as a side dish with frittata.

NUTRITIONAL INFORMATION:
Per Serving (excluding unknown items): 250 Calories; 11g Fat (38.6% calories from fat); 24g Protein; 14g Carbohydrate; 4g Dietary Fiber; Vegetable; 1/2 Fruit; 1 Fat; 0 Other Carbohydrates.

Lunch | (*phase III*)

(Hearty Black Bean Soup)

Serving : 4

1	lb black beans, soaked
2	medium onions – chopped
2	small carrots – chopped
1	celery stalk – chopped
4	cups of water
4	tsp extra virgin olive oil
1	large onion – chopped
4	cloves garlic – finely chopped
½	tsp dried oregano
½	tsp ground cumin
1	tsp soy sauce
1	tbsp fresh lemon juice

DIRECTIONS

Simmer beans in water till soft.

Sauté onions, celery & carrots in olive oil. Add garlic, cumin & soy sauce. Stir for 5 minutes.

Drain about 1/2 cup water from beans and add it to the sauté.

Cook over a low heat for 40 minutes.

Add vegetables to the beans.

Cook for another 30 minutes. Add more water if necessary.

Chicken and Summer Vegetable Broth

Serves : 4

2 quarts chicken stock

½ eggplant – diced

1 zucchini – diced

1 yellow squash – diced

1 red bell pepper – diced

½ cup Roma tomatoes – diced

½ cup green beans

½ cup lentils

1 bay leaf, whole

salt and pepper to taste

1 tbsp fresh basil – chopped

1 tsp fresh parsley – chopped

1 tsp fresh thyme – chopped

DIRECTIONS

Simmer lentils and bay leaf in chicken stock for 40 minutes.

Add remaining ingredients and simmer for 15 minutes.

Add fresh herbs and serve immediately.

NUTRITIONAL INFORMATION:

Per Serving (excluding unknown items): 171 Calories; 1g Fat (5.9% calories from fat); 11g Protein; 26g Carbohydrate; 11g Dietary Fiber; 0mg Cholesterol; 4304mg Sodium. Exchanges: 1 Grain(Starch); 1/2 Lean Meat; 2 Vegetable.

Dinner | (*phase III*)

Black Beans with Herb-Marinated Chicken and Marinated-Roasted Peppers

Serves : 4

2	red bell peppers, roasted, peeled, seeded, and sliced
1	green bell pepper, roasted, peeled, seeded, and sliced
1	yellow bell pepper, roasted, peeled, seeded, and sliced
3	cups black beans, cooked
2	chicken breasts, julienned into strips
3	tbsp lemon juice
1	tbsp fresh oregano, chopped
2	tbsp cilantro, chopped
1	tsp chili powder
1	tsp cumin
2	tbsp olive oil
$\frac{1}{3}$	cup pine nuts, toasted
2	cups chicken broth
	salt and pepper to taste

DIRECTIONS

Marinate Chicken Breast:
Combine half of the olive oil, oregano, cilantro, and lemon juice, and add all of the chili powder and cumin.

Let stand in refrigerator for 20 minutes, then drain marinade.

Heat remaining olive oil in a sauté pan over high heat. Sauté chicken breast strips until cooked through.

Add beans and bell peppers, pine nuts, and chicken broth, and heat through until peppers are slightly cooked, about 2 minutes. Remove from heat, stir in remaining fresh herbs, and serve.

NUTRITIONAL INFORMATION:

Per Serving (excluding unknown items): 252 Calories; 7g Fat (24.6% calories from fat); 9g Protein; 40g Carbohydrate; 4g Dietary Fiber; 107mg Cholesterol; 61mg Sodium. Exchanges: 1 1/2 Lean Meat; 1/2 Fruit; 0 Non-Fat Milk; 1 Fat; 1/2 Other Carbohydrates.

Mahi Mahi Satay with Lemongrass Brown Rice, Snow Peas, and Ponzu Dipping Sauce

Serves : 4

4	4-oz portions Mahi Mahi, cut into thin strips and skewered
1	cup ponzu
2	tbsp honey
1	tbsp cilantro, chopped
1	tsp ginger, minced
1	tsp scallion, minced
1	tsp garlic, minced
1	tsp sambal (asian hot sauce available at supermarkets)
1	tbsp sesame oil
⅔	cup brown rice, short grain
3	cups chicken broth
1	tbsp scallion, chopped
1	tbsp lemongrass, minced
2	cups snow peas
2	tbsp olive oil
1	tbsp soy sauce

DIRECTIONS

To make ponzu :
Combine ponzu, honey, cilantro, ginger, scallion, garlic, Sambal, and sesame oil.
In a pot, combine rice, broth, scallion, and lemongrass. Bring to a boil, reduce heat, covered, and simmer for approximately 45 minutes or until rice is cooked.

Marinate mahi mahi in ¼ of the ponzu dipping sauce for 10 minutes.

Place on hot grill and cook for approximately 1 ½ minutes per side.

Heat olive oil in a wok or sauté pan over high heat.

When oil begins to smoke, add snow peas and stir fry for 2 minutes, add soy sauce, mix in, remove from heat, and serve.

Serve skewers over rice and snow peas with ponzu dipping sauce on the side.

NUTRITIONAL INFORMATION:

Per Serving (excluding unknown items): 374 Calories; 12g Fat (29.8% calories from fat); 25g Protein; 39g Carbohydrate; 2g Dietary Fiber; 49mg Cholesterol; 1934mg Sodium. Exchanges: 1 1/2 Grain(Starch); 2 1/2 Lean Meat; 1 Vegetable; 2 Fat; 1/2 Other Carbohydrates.

Chicken Marsala with Brown Rice Risotto, Sautéed Haricot Verts with Marinated Tomatoes

Serves : 4

2	chicken breasts, sliced horizontally in 3 – 4 pc.
¼	cup whole wheat flour
¼	cup olive oil
1	ea bay leaf
2	tbsp dry marsala
1 ½	cups chicken broth, warm
1	cup mushrooms, sliced
	salt and pepper to taste
2	cups haricot verts (thin french string beans)
2	tsp olive oil
⅔	cup short grain brown rice
2 ⅔	cups water
¼	cup onion, diced
1	tsp olive oil
1	tbsp white wine
1	tbsp parmesan
1	tsp extra virgin olive oil
3	cups chicken stock
4	roma tomatoes, sliced ¼ inch thick
2	tbsp balsamic vinegar
1	tsp fresh oregano, chopped
1	tbsp fresh basil, cut into chiffonade (thin strips)
1	tsp extra virgin olive oil
	salt and pepper to taste

DIRECTIONS

In a saucepot, heat 2 tablespoons olive oil and 2 tablespoons of whole wheat flour and cook over medium heat until golden brown (this creates a nutty paste called a roux). Add mushrooms, cook for 3 minutes, and add marsala, cook for 1 minute. Add chicken broth and bay leaf, and simmer for 20 minutes.

Dredge chicken breast strips in remaining whole wheat flour. Heat 3 tablespoons olive oil in a sauté pan over high heat and add chicken until cooked through. Drain oil from pan. Add marsala sauce and warm through, but do not continue to cook the chicken breast or it will become overcooked.

To make Haricots verts:
Heat olive oil in a sauté pan over medium high heat. When oil is hot, add haricots verts and stir fry for 3 minutes, remove from heat, and serve.

To make Risotto:
Heat olive oil in saucepot, heat olive oil over medium, add onion and rice and sweat for 2 minutes. Add white wine and cook for 1 minute, then add 1 cup chicken stock. Stir rice frequently. As liquid is absorbed and the bottom of the pan is visible, add another cup of stock, repeating until all stock is absorbed, approximately 45 minutes. Drizzle with extra virgin olive oil and add parmesan if using.

To marinate Tomatoes:
Combine all ingredients.

NUTRITIONAL INFORMATION:

Per Serving (excluding unknown items): 374 Calories; 12g Fat (29.8% calories from fat); 25g Protein; 39g Carbohydrate; 2g Dietary Fiber; 49mg Cholesterol, 1934mg Sodium. Exchanges. 1 1/2 Grain(Starch), 2 1/2 Lean Meat; 1 Vegetable; 2 Fat; 1/2 Other Carbohydrates.

(Grilled Chicken Breast with Lentils, Creamless Cauliflower Gratin, and Jus)

Serves : 4

Marinade :

2	tbsp fresh lemon juice
2	tsp fresh oregano, chopped
4	tbsp fresh basil, cut into chiffonade (thin strips)
1	clove garlic
1	tbsp extra virgin olive oil
1 ½	cups dry lentils (recommend french lentils)
1	tbsp carrots, peeled and diced
1	tbsp celery, peeled and diced
1	tbsp yellow onion, peeled and diced
1	tsp garlic, minced
1	tbsp mushrooms, diced
1	tbsp olive oil,
2	tbsp red wine
2 ½	cups chicken stock
1	bay leaf
	salt and pepper to taste

Cauliflower Gratin :

1 head cauliflower, sliced into
     approximately ¼ inch thick pieces
½ yellow onion, julienned
1 tbsp olive oil
1 clove garlic, minced
1 tbsp white wine
1 tbsp parsley, chopped
2 tsp fresh thyme, chopped
1 ½ cups chicken stock
1 tbsp parmesan (optional)
  salt and pepper to taste

jus :

2 tsp olive oil
1 tbsp carrots, peeled and diced
1 tbsp celery, peeled and diced
1 tbsp yellow onion, peeled
    and diced
½ tsp garlic
1 tbsp white wine
2 ½ cups chicken stock
1 bay leaf
  salt and pepper to taste

DIRECTIONS

Combine marinade ingredients, add chicken, and let stand in refrigerator for 20 minutes. Drain marinade.

Lentils :
(double in size when cooked) Over medium heat, sweat lentils, carrots, celery, onion, garlic, and mushrooms in olive oil. Add red wine and cook for 2 minutes. Add chicken stock and bay leaf. Simmer until tender and liquid is absorbed, approximately 60-90 minutes. Remove bay leaf and serve.

Cauliflower Gratin :
In a sauté pan, heat olive oil over medium-low heat, add onion, and cook until soft and caramelized, approximately 4 minutes. Add cauliflower and sweat for approximately 2 minutes. Add garlic and cook for approximately 30 seconds. Add wine and cook for approximately 1 minute. Add chicken stock, stir in parsley and thyme. Cover with foil and bake in 400° F oven for 20 minutes. Remove foil, sprinkle with parmesan (if using) and place under broiler for approximately 5 minutes to brown on top.

Jus :
Over medium heat, sweat carrots, celery, onion, and garlic in olive oil. Add white wine and cook for 2 minutes. Add chicken stock and bay leaf. Simmer for 20 minutes and strain.

NUTRITIONAL INFORMATION:

Per Serving (excluding unknown items): 556 Calories; 15g Fat (25.5% calories from fat); 50g Protein; 49g Carbohydrate; 24g Dietary Fiber; 68mg Cholesterol; 3593mg Sodium. Exchanges: 3 Grain(Starch); 5 1/2 Lean Meat; 1 Vegetable; 0 Fruit; 2 1/2 Fat.

PHASE IV | Sample Recipes

Breakfast | (*phase IV*)

Recipes on the go!

- 2 (4-inch) pancakes
  1 tbsp syrup
  ½ cup of strawberries
  1 cup low-fat milk or
    orange or apple juice

- 1 mini bagel
  2 tsp jelly
  1 tbsp cream cheese
  1 cup low-fat milk or
    orange or apple juice

➤➤

- 2 slices whole-wheat bread, toasted
  1 egg, scrambled
  1 tsp butter
  1 slice American cheese
  1 cup low-fat milk
  1 medium banana

- 2 low-fat waffles
  1 tsp syrup
  1 cup fresh orange juice
  1 cup low-fat yogurt

Blueberry Buckwheat Pancakes with Strawberry and Orange Compote

Serves : 4

4 oz buckwheat flour

1 oz granulated sugar substitute
   (splenda recommended)

2 tsp baking powder

½ tsp salt

2 large eggs, beaten

8 oz nonfat milk

½ cup blueberries

1 tbsp olive oil

1 cup strawberries, sliced

½ cup orange juice

1 tbsp granulated sugar substitute

DIRECTIONS

To make orange compote :
Combine orange juice, strawberries, and sugar substitute and cook over low heat for 25 minutes. Let stand until warm or room temperature

To make pancakes :
Sift first four ingredients together into a medium mixing bowl. Add milk, eggs, and blueberries to dry ingredients. Do not overmix. Batter should remain slightly lumpy. Heat olive oil in nonstick pan or griddle over medium heat. Spoon about 2 oz. Of pancake batter onto griddle for about 2 minutes or until edges become opaque and air bubbles on surface of pancakes begin to pop. Flip pancakes and cook for another 2 minutes. Serve warm and drizzled with compote.

NUTRITIONAL INFORMATION:

Per Serving (excluding unknown items): 252 Calories; 7g Fat (24.6% calories from fat); 9g Protein; 40g Carbohydrate; 4g Dietary Fiber; 107mg Cholesterol; 614mg Sodium. Exchanges: 1 1/2 Grain(Starch); 1/2 Lean Meat; 1/2 Fruit; 0 Non-Fat Milk; 1 Fat; 1/2 Other Carbohydrates.

Banana Stuffed Whole Wheat French Toast with Mango Compote

Serves : 4

8 slices whole wheat bread

3 bananas, sliced thinly
   on the bias

2 cups nonfat milk

1 large egg

1 tbsp granulated sugar
   substitute
   (splenda recommended)

1 tsp cinnamon

2 tbsp olive oil

2 mangos, peeled, pitted,
   and diced

3 tbsp granulated sugar substitute
   (splenda recommended)

DIRECTIONS

To make mango compote :
Combine mangos and sugar substitute and cook
over low heat for 20 minutes. Let stand until
warm or room temperature.

Mix milk, egg, sugar substitute, and cinnamon.

Heat olive oil in nonstick pan or griddle over medium heat.

Distribute banana slices on four slices of bread,
then gently press remaining four slices of bread on
top of each bottom slice.

Dip bread in milk and egg mixture, and cook over
medium heat for about 3 minutes per side,
or until golden.

Spoon mango compote over each serving.

NUTRITIONAL INFORMATION:

Per Serving (excluding unknown items): 399 Calories; 11g Fat (23.9%
calories from fat); 12g Protein; 67g Carbohydrate; 7g Dietary Fiber;
55mg Cholesterol; 402mg Sodium. Exchanges: 1 1/2 Grain(Starch); 0
Lean Meat; 2 Fruit; 1/2 Non-Fat Milk; 2 Fat; 1/2 Other Carbohydrates.

Egg White Omelet with Low Fat Cheddar Cheese and Fresh Herbs

Serves : 4

18	egg whites
2	tbsp olive oil
1 ½	cups cheddar cheese, lowfat – shredded
1	tsp fresh thyme – chopped
1	tsp fresh parsley – chopped
1	tsp fresh chives – chopped
½	cup strawberries – sliced
	salt and pepper to taste

DIRECTIONS

Whisk together egg whites, herbs, and salt and pepper.

In a nonstick omelet pan, heat 1/4 of the oil and pour in 1/4 of the egg white mixtures.

Cook until set, stirring constantly with rubber spatula.

Stir in cheese, fold over, and serve with side of strawberries.

NUTRITIONAL INFORMATION:

Per Serving (excluding unknown items): 215 Calories; 10g Fat (42.3% calories from fat); 26g Protein; 4g Carbohydrate; 1g Dietary Fiber; 9mg Cholesterol; 506mg Sodium. Exchanges: 0 Grain(Starch); 3 1/2 Lean Meat; 0 Vegetable; 0 Fruit; 1 1/2 Fat.

Dinner | (*phase IV*)

Ahi Fish Tacos with Roasted Poblano Guacamole

Serves : 4

4	tortillas, whole wheat 96% fat free flour
10	oz tuna steak – sliced 1/2" thick
¼	tsp chili powder
¼	tsp cumin
¼	tsp dried oregano
¼	tsp salt and pepper to taste
¼	tsp cayenne pepper
¼	tsp cinnamon
1	tbsp olive oil
1	cup iceberg lettuce – shredded
1	red bell pepper – julienned
½	cup red onion – julienned
¼	cup fresh cilantro – chopped
1	tbsp rice wine vinegar
1	tbsp lemon juice
2	tbsp hot sauce
1	small poblano pepper – roasted, peeled, and diced
1	small avocado – peeled and chopped
1	tsp lemon juice
1	tsp minced garlic
1	tbsp roma tomato – diced
1	tbsp red onion – diced
1	tbsp minced cilantro
	salt and pepper to taste

DIRECTIONS

Combine chili powder, cumin, dried oregano, salt and pepper, cayenne pepper, and cinnamon, and sprinkle on fish to season.

Sear tuna in olive oil over very high heat (tuna should remain slightly pink in center). Combine vinegar, lemon juice, and hot sauce (any favorite variety) and toss with lettuce, bell pepper, red onion, and cilantro.

For guacamole, combine poblano pepper, avocado, lemon juice, garlic, tomato, red onion, salt and pepper and cilantro and blend well.

Place fish and vegetable mixture into tortillas and cut tacos in half.

Serve two halves per serving. Garnish with guacamole.

NUTRITIONAL INFORMATION:

Per Serving (excluding unknown items): 384 Calories; 17g Fat (39.5% calories from fat); 23g Protein; 37g Carbohydrate; 5g Dietary Fiber; 27mg Cholesterol; 695mg Sodium. Exchanges: 0 Grain(Starch); 2 1/2 Lean Meat; 1 Vegetable; 0 Fruit; 2 Fat; 0 Other Carbohydrates.

Roasted Chicken Breast with Brown Saffron Risotto, Oven Dried Tomatoes, and Basil/Mint Jus

Serves : 4

Chicken breast :

2   chicken breasts, boneless
and skinless, approx. 7-8 oz. each
salt and pepper to taste
**roast chicken breast in a
400° F oven until done,
approximately 10 minutes.
Let cool and slice into strips.*

Basil/Mint Broth :

2   tsp olive oil
1   tbsp carrots, peeled
and diced
1   tbsp celery, peeled
and diced
1   tbsp yellow onion, peeled
and diced
½   tsp garlic
1   tbsp white wine
2 ½   cups of chicken stock
1   bay leaf
2   sprigs fresh basil
2   sprigs fresh mint
salt and pepper to taste

DIRECTIONS

To make basil/mint broth :
Over medium heat, sweat carrots, celery, onion, and garlic in olive oil.

Add white wine and cook for 2 minutes.

Add chicken stock, basil, mint, and bay leaf.

Simmer for 20 minutes. Strain.

Oven-dried Tomatoes :
16   Roma tomatoes, quartered
     (see shortcut substitution below)
1   tbsp olive oil

DIRECTIONS

To make oven- dried tomatoes :
Drizzle tomatoes with olive oil.

Place in 225 F oven for 4 hours and remove.

Let cool. (Note substitution: can use sun dried tomatoes, simmered in water for 10 minutes and drained, then tossed with olive oil)

Risotto :

2   cups short grain brown rice

2   tsp olive oil

2   tbsp yellow onion, peeled and diced

1   tbsp white wine

7   cups chicken stock, hot

1   tbsp saffron

1   tsp extra virgin olive oil

    salt and pepper to taste

1   tbsp parmesan (optional)

DIRECTIONS

To make risotto :
Tip: Keep chicken stock simmering in a separate pot next to the risotto. Heat olive oil in saucepot, heat olive oil over medium, add onion and rice and sweat for 2 minutes.

Add white wine and cook for 1 minute, then add 1 cup chicken stock and saffron. Stir rice frequently.

As liquid is absorbed and the bottom of the pan is visible, add another cup of stock, repeating until all stock is absorbed, approximately 45 minutes.

Drizzle with extra virgin olive oil and add parmesan if using.

To serve :
Spoon risotto into bowls and add tomatoes and chicken.

NUTRITIONAL INFORMATION:

Per Serving (excluding unknown items): 721 Calories; 15g Fat (19.6% calories from fat); 41g Protein; 99g Carbohydrate; 7g Dietary Fiber; 68mg Cholesterol; 5228mg Sodium. Exchanges: 5 Grain(Starch); 4 Lean Meat; 4 1/2 Vegetable; 2 Fat.

SNACKS:

- ⅓ cup plain low-fat yogurt dip and 2 cups raw vegetables

- cashews (10)

- 2 graham cracker squares and 2 tsp low-sugar jelly

- 1 low-fat Granola bar

- 15 grapes and ½ cup of low fat milk

- ½ cup of plain low-fat yogurt

- 2 tbsp raisins and 10 peanuts

- 1 small brownie

- 2 gingersnaps and ½ oz cheddar cheese

- 1 ½ cups of baby carrots

- 2 chocolate chip cookies-small

- tortilla chips, fat-free (15-20)

- ½ small pack of licorice

- Almonds (10-14)

- Jell-O Smoothie snacks (1 snack)

- 4 animal crackers and 1 small orange

- popcorn, air popped (3 cups, no butter!)

- 2 rice cakes topped with 1 tsp peanut butter

- 1 cup unsweetened applesauce

- saltine crackers (7)

- 1 medium banana, frozen

- 8 halves dried apricots and ½ cup skim milk

- sunflower seeds (2 tbsp)

- sherbert (½ cup)

- ½ cup sugar free chocolate pudding made with low-fat milk with 2 tbsp whipped topping

- Melba toast (4 slices)

- 6 saltine-type crackers topped with 2 tsp low-sugar jelly

"For those readers who may lack the time or ability to prepare the recipes in this book, or for those who may enjoy an additional selection of recipes consistent with Dr. Ian's nutritional guidelines, you may contact Big City Chefs at the number provided at the beginning of this chapter. Big City Chefs staffs professionally-trained personal chefs in major metropolitan regions nationwide, providing personalized menu planning and in-home preparation of one to two weeks of meals per visit."

APPENDIX

BODY MASS INDEX (*BMI*)

Height	18	19	20	21	22	23	24	25	26	27	28	29	30	31	32	33	34	35	36	37	38	39
									Body Weight (pounds)													
4'10"	86	91	96	100	105	110	115	119	124	129	134	138	143	148	153	158	162	167	172	177	181	186
4'11"	89	94	99	104	109	114	119	124	128	133	138	143	148	153	158	163	168	173	178	183	188	193
5'0"	92	97	102	107	112	118	123	128	133	138	143	148	153	158	163	168	174	179	184	189	194	199
5'1"	95	100	106	111	116	122	127	132	137	143	148	153	158	164	169	174	180	185	190	195	201	206
5'2"	98	104	109	115	120	126	131	136	142	147	153	158	164	169	175	180	186	191	196	202	207	213
5'3"	102	107	113	118	124	130	135	141	146	152	158	163	169	175	180	186	191	197	203	208	214	220
5'4"	105	110	116	122	128	134	140	145	151	157	163	169	174	180	186	192	197	204	209	215	221	227
5'5"	108	114	120	126	132	138	144	150	156	162	168	174	180	186	192	198	204	210	216	222	228	234
5'6"	112	118	124	130	136	142	148	155	161	167	173	179	186	192	198	204	210	216	223	229	235	241
5'7"	115	121	127	134	140	146	153	159	166	172	178	185	191	198	204	211	217	223	230	236	242	249
5'8"	118	125	131	138	144	151	158	165	171	177	184	190	197	203	210	216	223	230	236	243	249	256
5'9"	122	128	135	142	149	155	162	169	176	182	189	196	203	209	216	223	230	236	243	250	257	263
5'10"	126	132	139	146	153	160	167	174	181	188	195	202	209	216	222	229	236	243	250	257	264	271
5'11"	129	136	143	150	157	165	172	179	186	193	200	208	215	222	229	236	243	250	257	265	272	279
6'0"	132	140	147	154	162	169	177	184	191	199	206	213	221	228	235	242	250	258	265	272	279	287
6'1"	136	144	151	159	166	174	182	189	197	204	212	219	227	235	242	250	257	265	272	280	288	295
6'2"	141	148	155	163	171	179	186	194	202	210	218	225	233	241	249	256	264	272	280	287	295	303
6'3"	144	152	160	168	176	184	192	200	208	216	224	232	240	248	256	264	272	279	287	295	303	311
6'4"	148	156	164	172	180	189	197	205	213	221	230	238	246	254	263	271	279	287	295	304	312	320
6'5"	151	160	168	176	185	193	202	210	218	227	235	244	252	261	269	277	286	294	303	311	319	328
6'6"	155	164	172	181	190	198	207	216	224	233	241	250	259	267	276	284	293	302	310	319	328	336

UNDERWEIGHT	HEALTHY WEIGHT	OVERWEIGHT	OBESE
(<18.5)	(18.5–24.9)	(25–29.9)	(≥30)

Find your height along the left-hand column and look across the row until you find the number that is closest to your weight. The number at the top of that column identifies your BMI.

Source: From A. Must, G. E. Dallal, and W. H. Dietz, "Reference Data for Obesity: 85th and 95th Percentiles of Body Mass Index (wt/ht2) and Triceps Skinfold Thickness." *American Journal of Clinical Nutrition* 53 (1991): 839–846. Adapted with permission by the *American Journal of Clinical Nutrition*, © American Journal of Clinical Nutrition, American Society for Clinical Nutrition.

FIBER CONTENT OF FOODS

To consume more fiber, eat more whole fruits and vegetables, whole grains, and beans. Nuts are also rich in fiber, but they are energy dense, so eat them in small amounts. Use the following list to guide your food choices. It is adapted from research conducted by the Tufts University School of Medicine in Boston and published in the *Tufts Health & Nutrition Letter*.

FRUITS*	GRAMS OF FIBER
Apple (with skin)	4
Banana	3
Blueberries, ½ cup	2
Cantaloupe, 1 cup diced	1
Dates, ⅛ cup dry, chopped	2
Grapefruit, ½	2
Grapes, 1 cup	2
Nectarine (with skin)	2
Orange	3
Peach (with skin)	2
Pear (with skin)	4
Plum (with skin)	1
Prunes (dried), 10	2
Raisins, ⅛ cup	1
Raspberries, ½ cup	4
Strawberries, ½ cup	2
Watermelon, 1 cup diced	1

VEGETABLES†	GRAMS OF FIBER
Broccoli, ½ cup cooked, chopped	2
Broccoli, ½ cup chopped	1

*All values are for 1 medium-size fruit unless otherwise indicated.

†All values are for raw, uncooked vegetables unless otherwise indicated.

Brussels sprouts, ½ cup cooked	3
Carrot, 1 medium	2
Carrots, ½ cup cooked	3
Cauliflower, ½ cup cooked	2
Celery, 1 stalk	1
Corn, ½ cup cooked	2
Cucumber, ½ cup sliced	0.5
French fries, 1 small (2.5 ounces) serving	2
Green beans, ½ cup cooked (frozen)	2
Iceberg lettuce, 1 cup shredded	1
Peas, ½ cup cooked (frozen)	4
Peppers, ½ cup chopped	1
Potato, baked, with skin	5
Potato, baked, without skin	2
Potato, ½ cup mashed	2
Romaine lettuce, 1 cup shredded	1
Spinach, ½ cup chopped	1
Spinach, ½ cup cooked (frozen)	3
Sweet potato, baked with skin	3
Tomato, 1 medium	1

GRAINS, LEGUMES* (BEANS, CHICKPEAS, LENTILS, LIMA BEANS), AND NUTS

	GRAMS OF FIBER
Black beans, ½ cup	8
Bread, 1 slice, white	1
Bread, 1 slice, whole-wheat	2
Bran muffin, 1 medium	3

*Values are for canned or cooked beans.

(Grains, Legumes, and Nuts, continued)	GRAMS OF FIBER
Chickpeas, ½ cup	5
Kidney beans, ½ cup	7
Lentils, ½ cup	8
Lima beans, ½ cup	6
Oatmeal, 1 cup cooked	4
Pasta, ½ cup cooked	1
Peanuts, ½ cup	6
Peanut butter, 2 tablespoons, chunky	2
Popcorn, 3 cups air-popped	2
Rice, 1 cup cooked, white	1
Rice, 1 cup cooked, brown	2
Sesame seeds, 2 tablespoons	1
Sunflower seeds, ⅛ cup	2
Tortilla chips, 1 cup (1.5 oz.)	1
Walnuts, ¼ cup chopped	2
Wheat germ, ¼ cup	4

GLYCEMIC INDEX OF SAMPLE FOODS

BEANS

baby lima   32
baked   43
black   30
brown   38
butter   31
chickpeas   33
kidney   27
lentil   30
navy   38
pinto   42
red lentils   27
split peas   32
soy   18

BREADS

bagel   72
croissant   67
kaiser roll   73
pita   57
pumpernickel   49
rye   64
rye, dark   76
rye, whole   50
white   72
whole wheat   72
waffles   76

CEREALS

All-Bran   44
Bran Chex   58
Cheerios   74
corn bran   75
Corn Chex   83
cornflakes   83
Cream of Wheat   66
Crispix   87
Frosted Flakes   55
Grape-Nuts   67
Grape-Nuts Flakes   80
Life   66
muesli   60
NutriGrain   66
oatmeal   49
oatmeal 1 min.   66
puffed wheat   74
puffed rice   90
rice bran   19
Rice Chex   89
Rice Krispies   82
Shredded Wheat   69
Special K   54
Swiss muesli   60
Team   82
Total   76

COOKIES

graham crackers   74
oatmeal   55
shortbread   64
vanilla wafers   77

CRACKERS

Kavli Norwegian   71
rice cakes   82
rye   63
saltine   72
stoned wheat thins   67
water crackers   78

DESSERTS

FRUIT

GRAINS

JUICES

MILK PRODUCTS

PASTA

vermicelli   35
vermicelli, rice   58

SWEETS

honey   58
jelly beans   80

Life Savers   70
M&M's chocolate peanut   33
Skittles   70
Snickers   41

Source: The Diabetes Mall, www.diabetes-mall.com

HOW TO READ A FOOD LABEL

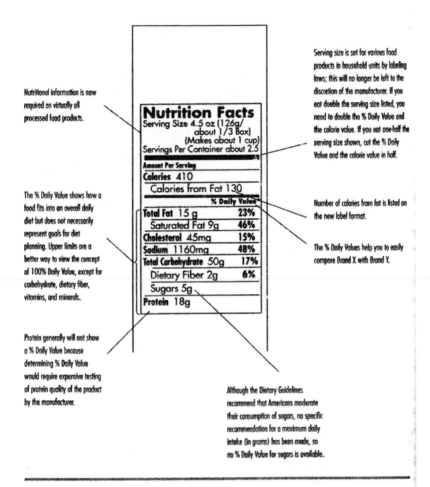

Nutritional information is now required on virtually all processed food products.

The % Daily Value shows how a food fits into an overall daily diet but does not necessarily represent goals for diet planning. Upper limits are a better way to view the concept of 100% Daily Value, except for carbohydrate, dietary fiber, vitamins, and minerals.

Protein generally will not show a % Daily Value because determining % Daily Value would require expensive testing of protein quality of the product by the manufacturer.

Serving size is set for various food products in household units by labeling laws; this will no longer be left to the discretion of the manufacturer. If you eat double the serving size listed, you need to double the % Daily Value and the calorie value. If you eat one-half the serving size shown, cut the % Daily Value and the calorie value in half.

Number of calories from fat is listed on the new label format.

The % Daily Values help you to easily compare Brand X with Brand Y.

Although the Dietary Guidelines recommend that Americans moderate their consumption of sugars, no specific recommendation for a maximum daily intake (in grams) has been made, so no % Daily Value for sugars is available.

Nutrition Facts
Serving Size 4.5 oz (126g/ about 1/3 Box) (Makes about 1 cup)
Servings Per Container about 2.5

Amount Per Serving

Calories 410   Calories from Fat 130

	% Daily Value
Total Fat 15 g	23%
Saturated Fat 9g	46%
Cholesterol 45mg	15%
Sodium 1160mg	48%
Total Carbohydrate 50g	17%
Dietary Fiber 2g	6%
Sugars 5g	
Protein 18g	

The Nutrition Facts panel on a current food label. The box is broken into two parts: A is the top, and B is the bottom. The % Daily Value listed on the label is the percentage of the generally accepted amount of a nutrient needed daily that is present in 1 serving of the product. You can use the % Daily Values to compare your diet with current nutrition recommendations for certain diet components. Let's consider dietary fiber. Assume that you consume 2,000 kcal. per day, which is the energy intake corresponding to the % Daily Values listed on labels. If the total % Daily Value for dietary fiber in all the foods you eat in one day adds up to 100%, your diet meets the recommendations for dietary fiber.

Many vitamin and mineral amounts no longer need to be listed on the nutrition label. Only Vitamin A, Vitamin C, calcium, and iron remain. The interest in or risk of deficiencies of the other vitamins and minerals is deemed too low to warrant inclusion.

Some % Daily Value standards, such as grams of total fat, increase as energy intake increases. The % Daily Values on the label are based on a 2,000-kcal. diet. This is important to note if you don't consume at least 2,000 kcal. per day.

Labels on larger packages may list the number of calories per gram of fat, carbohydrate, and protein.

Ingredients, listed in descending order by weight, will appear here or in another place on the package. The sources of some ingredients, such as certain flavorings, will be stated by name to help people better identify ingredients that they avoid for health, religious, or other reasons.

| Vitamin A 10% • Vitamin C 0% |
| Calcium 30% •Iron 15% |

Percent Daily Values are based on a 2,000 calorie diet. Your daily values may be higher or lower depending on your calorie needs:

		Calories: 2,000	2,500
Total Fat	Less than	65g	80g
Sat Fat	Less than	20g	25g
Cholest	Less than	300mg	300mg
Sodium	Less than	2,400mg	2,400mg
Total Carb		300g	375g
Fiber		25g	30g

Calories per gram:
Fat 9 • Carbohydrate 4
• Protein 4

INGREDIENTS: WATER, ENRICHED MACARONI [ENRICHED FLOUR [NIACIN, FERROUS SULFATE (IRON), THIAMINE MONONITRATE AND RIBOFLAVIN], EGG WHITE], FLOUR, CHEDDAR CHEESE (MILK, CHEESE CULTURE, SALT, ENZYME), SPICES, MARGARINE (PARTIALLY HYDROGENATED SOYBEAN OIL, WATER, SOY LECITHIN, MONO- AND DIGLYCERIDES, BETA CARO-TENE FOR COLOR, VITAMIN A PALMITATE), AND MALTODEXTRIN.

Source: Wardlaw, Gordon M., *Contemporary Nutrition*, 4th ed. (New York: McGraw Hill Companies, Inc., 2000).

CALORIC EXPENDITURE
DURING VARIOUS ACTIVITIES

ACTIVITY	CAL/MIN*
Sleeping	1.2
Resting in bed	1.3
Sitting, normally	1.3
Sitting, reading	1.3
Lying, quietly	1.3
Sitting, eating	1.5
Sitting, playing cards	1.5
Standing, normally	1.5
Classwork, lecture (listening)	1.7
Conversing	1.8
Personal toilet	2.0
Sitting, writing	2.6
Standing, light activity	2.6
Washing and dressing	2.6
Washing and shaving	2.6
Driving a car	2.8
Washing clothes	3.1
Walking indoors	3.1
Shining shoes	3.2
Making bed	3.4
Dressing	3.4
Showering	3.4
Driving motorcycle	3.4

*Depends on efficiency and body size. Add 10 percent for each 15 lb. over 150; subtract 10 percent for each 15 lb. under 150.

ACTIVITY	CAL/MIN
Metalworking	3.5
House painting	3.5
Cleaning windows	3.7
Carpentry	3.8
Farming chores	3.8
Sweeping floors	3.9
Plastering walls	4.1
Repairing trucks and automobiles	4.2
Ironing clothes	4.2
Farming, planting, hoeing, raking	4.7
Mixing cement	4.7
Mopping floors	4.9
Repaving roads	5.0
Gardening, weeding	5.6
Stacking lumber	5.8
Sawing with chain saw	6.2
Working with stone, masonry	6.3
Working with pick and shovel	6.7
Farming, haying, plowing with horse	6.7
Shoveling (miners)	6.8
Shoveling snow	7.5
Walking down stairs	7.1
Chopping wood	7.5
Sawing with crosscut saw	7.5–10.5
Tree felling (ax)	8.4–12.7
Gardening, digging	8.6
Walking up stairs	10.0–18.0
Playing pool or billiards	1.8
Canoeing, 2.5 mph–4.0 mph	3.0–7.0

ACTIVITY	CAL/MIN
Playing volleyball, recreational to competitive	3.5–8.0
Golfing, foursome to twosome	3.7–5.0
Pitching horseshoes	3.8
Playing baseball (except pitcher)	4.7
Playing Ping-Pong or table tennis	4.9–7.0
Practicing calisthenics	5.0
Rowing, pleasure to vigorous	5.0–15.0
Cycling, easy to hard	5.0–15.0
Skating, recreational to vigorous	5.0–15.0
Practicing archery	5.2
Playing badminton, recreational to competitive	5.2–10.0
Playing basketball, half or full court (more for fast break)	6.0–9.0
Bowling (while active)	7.0
Playing tennis, recreational to competitive	7.0–11.0
Waterskiing	8.0
Playing soccer	9.0
Snowshoeing (2.5 mph)	9.0
Slide board	9.0–13.0
Playing handball or squash	10.0
Mountain climbing	10.0–15.0
Skipping rope	10.0–15.0
Practicing judo or karate	13.0
Playing football (while active)	13.3
Wrestling	14.4
Skiing	
Moderate to steep	8.0–20.0

ACTIVITY	CAL/MIN
Downhill racing	16.5
Cross-country; 3–10 mph	9.0–20.0
Swimming	
Leisurely	6.0
Crawl, 25–50 yd/min.	6.0–12.5
Butterfly, 50 yd/min.	14.0
Backstroke, 25–50 yd/min.	6.0–12.5
Breaststroke, 25–50 yd/min.	6.0–12.5
Sidestroke, 40 yd/min.	11.0
Dancing	
Modern, moderate to vigorous	4.2–5.7
Ballroom, waltz to rumba	5.7–7.0
Square	7.7
Walking	
Road or field (3.5 mph)	5.6–7.0
Snow, hard to soft (2.5–3.5 mph)	10.0–20.0
Uphill, 15 percent grade (3.5 mph)	8.0–15.0
Downhill, 5–10 percent grade (2.5 mph)	3.5–3.7
15–20 percent grade (2.5 mph)	3.7–4.3
Hiking, 40-lb. pack (3.0 mph)	6.8
Running	
12-min. mile (5 mph)	10.0
8-min. mile (7.5 mph)	15.0
6-min. mile (10 mph)	20.0
5-min. mile (12 mph)	25.0

Source: Sharkey, Brian J., PhD., *Fitness and Health,* 4th ed. (Champaign: Human Kinetics, 1997).

BIBLIOGRAPHY

Books

Atkins, Robert C., M.D., *Dr. Atkin's Diet Revolution* (New York: Bantam, 1972).

Brody, Tom, *Nutritional Biochemistry*, 2nd ed (Academic Press, 1999).

Cooper, Kenneth H., M.D., M.PH., *The Aerobics Program for Total Well-Being* (New York: Bantam Books, 1982).

Hensrud, Donald D., M.D., *Mayo Clinic on Healthy Weight* (New York: Kensington Publishing Corporation, 2000).

Katch, Frank I., and McArdle, William D., *Introduction to Nutrition, Exercise, and Health*, 4th ed. (Baltimore: Lippincott Williams and Wilkins, 1988).

Mathews, Christopher K., and van Holde, K. E., *Biochemistry* (Redwood City, Calif.: Benjamin/Cummings Publishing Company, 1990).

McArdle, William D., Katch, Frank I., and Katch, Victor L., *Exercise Physiology: Energy, Nutrition, and Human Performance*, 4th ed. (New York: Lippincott Williams and Wilkins, 1996).

Paulsen, Barbara, *The Diet Advisor* (New York: Time-Life Books, 2000).

Rolls, Barbara, Ph.D., and Barnett, Robert, *Volumetrics Weight-Control Plan* (New York: HarperCollins, 2000).

Sears, Barry, Ph.D., *The Zone* (New York: HarperCollins, 1995).

Sharkey, Brian J., PhD., *Fitness and Health*, 4th ed. (Champaign: Human Kinetics, 1997).

Sizer, Frances, and Whitney, Eleanor, *Nutrition: Concepts and Controversies*, 8th ed. (Stamford: Wadsworth/Thomson Learning, 2000).

Steward, H. Leighton, Bethea, Morrison C., Nadrews, Samˇ S., Brennan, Ralph O., and Balart, Luis A. , *Sugar Busters!: Cut Sugar to Trim Fat* (New York: Ballantine, 1998).

Tarnower, Herman, and Baker, Samm Sinclair *Complete Scarsdale Medical Diet*

Plus Dr. Tarnower's Lifetime Keep-Slim Program (New York: Bantam Books, 1995).

Wardlaw, Gordon M., *Contemporary Nutrition: Issues and Insights,* 4th ed. (New York: The McGraw-Hill Companies, Inc., 2000).

Studies/Articles

The American Dietetics' Association Food and Nutrition Guide.

Willett, W.C., Dietz, W. H., and Colditz, G. A., "Guidelines for Healthy Weight," *New England Journal of Medicine* 341 (1999): 427–34.

National Institutes of Health, "Clinical Guidelines on the Identification, Evaluation, and Treatment of Overweight and Obesity in Adults" (September 1998).

U.S. Department of Health and Human Services, "Physical Activity and Health: A Report of the Surgeon General" (Atlanta, GA.: Centers for Disease Control and Prevention, National Center for Chronic Disease Prevention and Health Promotion, 1996).

Paffenbarger, R. S., Hyde, R. T., Wing, A. L., et al., "The Association of Changes in Physical-Activity Level and Other Lifestyle Characteristics with Mortality Among Men," *New England Journal of Medicine* 328, no. 8 (1993): 538–45.

Sherman, S. E., D'Agostino, R. B., Cobb, J. L., et al., "Physical Activity and Mortality in Women in the Framingham Heart Study," *American Heart Journal* 128, no. 5 (1994): 879–84.

Pate, R. R., Pratt, M., Blair, S. N., et al. "Physical Activity and Public Health: A Recommendation from the Centers for Disease Control and Prevention and the American College of Sports Medicine," *Journal of the American Medical Association* 273, no. 5 (1995): 402–407.

USDA and U.S. Department of Health and Human Services, *Dietary Guidelines for Americans,* 5th ed. (USDA Home and Garden Bulletin No. 232. Washington, D.C.: USDA, 2000).

USDA, *The Food Guide Pyramid* (USDA Home and Garden Bulletin No. 252. Washington, D.C.: USDA, 1992).

Flegal, K. M., Carroll, M.D., Kuczmarski, R. J., et al, "Overweight and Obesity in the United States: Prevalence and Trends, 1960–1994," *International Journal of Obesity* 22, no. 1 (1998): 39–47.

NIH, "Clinical Guideline on the Identification, Evaluation and Treatment of Overweight and Obesity in Adults—The Evidence Report," *Obesity Research* 6 (suppl. 2, 1998): 51S–209S.

PHS, *The Surgeon General's Report on Nutrition and Health* (DHHS Pub. No. [PHS] 88050210, Washington, D.C.: HHS, 1988).

ABOUT THE AUTHOR

Dr. Ian Smith is currently a medical contributor to ABC's nationally syndicated, "The View", a medical columnist for *Men's Health* magazine, and the medical/diet expert on VH1's "Celebrity Fit Club." Dr. Smith is also the host of the nationally syndicated radio show *Healthwise* on American Urban Radio Networks. He is the former medical correspondent for NBC News network and for NewsChannel 4 where he filed reports for NBC's "Nightly News" and the "Today" show as well as WNBC's various news broadcasts. He has written for various publications including *Time, Newsweek,* and the *New York Daily News,* and has been featured in several other publications including, *People, Essence, Ebony, Cosmopolitan,* and *University of Chicago Medicine on the Midway.*

Dr. Smith graduated from Harvard College with an AB and received a master's in science education from Columbia University. He attended Dartmouth Medical School and completed the last two years of his medical education and graduated from the University of Chicago Pritzker School of Medicine.

Dr. Smith is also the author of four books, the recently released *The Fat Smash Diet,* the critically acclaimed *The Blackbird Papers* **(2005 BCALA fiction Honor Book Award winner***), Dr. Ian Smith's Guide to Medical Websites* and *The Take-Control Diet.*

MY WEIGHT LOSS JOURNAL

160